I0421407

1 Weight Loss Plan,

2 Friends,

3 Weeks

Using the Buddy System to Fight Fat

April Paine and Stacey Wein

Copyright © 2013

All rights reserved

The information contained in this book is anecdotal and meant to serve as a guide of strategies that the authors have applied. Always check with a doctor before beginning any diet or physical exercise program. The authors make it clear that they are not doctors and cannot be held responsible for any adverse occurrence due to the anecdotal recommendations in this book. Reading this book and applying the strategies guarantees nothing. The authors have made all reasonable efforts to provide accurate information for the readers. The authors will not be held liable for any unintentional errors or side effects due to the use of the strategies suggested. By continuing to read this book, the reader accepts full responsibility.

No part of this book may be reproduced without the express written permission of the authors or their publisher. All rights reserved.

Dedication

To all the women and men out there who have ever looked for happiness at the bottom of a cookie jar. We hope you find it in friendship instead, as we did.

Note:

Outside of the authors, names have been changed to protect the privacy of the innocent (those we accused of stealing our last Oreos) and the not-so-innocent (those who tempted us with Oreos).

Be true to your work, your word and your friend.

-Henry David Thoreau

Contents

Introduction

Three weeks. Less time than it takes for your bikini wax to grow out. Three weeks. That's all the time it took for us to see that we were on to something good. We threw out our old diet books—turned our backs on the notion that we could shed pounds through the help of blood tests, raw food, too much protein, too little protein, pills, shakes and hypnosis. And we turned to something that costs nothing. Friendship.

We first bonded over pints of ice cream and deep-dish pizza during our first year of college. We put on the freshman 5, 10, 15 and 20 and throughout the next four years, lost and regained it a dozen times each. We knew that we needed to change our weight loss strategy when our thighs developed such distinct personalities that it became necessary to name them. Each of us desperately wanted to help the other change her unhealthy ways but we didn't know how to begin. It took us a decade apart, April in Manhattan and Stacey in Los Angeles, and countless trials with every weight loss remedy known to man and woman. But we finally figured out how to break free from the cycle of weight loss/weight gain and the best part is…we did it together!

If you want to learn how to play the guitar, you find an instructor and take lessons. If you want to learn how to skydive, you find a VERY good instructor, take lessons and jump. But, where do you go, who do you consult, if you want to learn how to lose weight and keep it off?

Your choices are endless; there are a variety of educated specialists to consult, like physical fitness trainers and nutritionists. There are well-established organizations to assist you, such as Weight Watchers and Jenny Craig. It seems every week there's a new radio spot for herbal remedies promising to "trap the fat" or quell your hunger so you'll eat less. There are exercise programs and diets too numerous to name, promoted by doctors and celebrities, each touting THEIR approach as YOUR answer to weight loss.

So, with all these choices, all these options, why has the number of obese people in America grown at alarming rates? Why do most women continue to admit they are dissatisfied with their bodies, and so many people suffer from some kind of eating disorder? Most diet programs fail, causing participants to gain back their lost pounds and then some. That's not encouraging.

Perhaps there are too many choices. It's overwhelming just to settle on a strategy. It's a challenge to commit to a program and stick with a plan when trying to conquer one of the toughest personal battles a person can face.

Enter your new best friends: Stacey & April. We want to introduce you to a powerful weight loss strategy. But we don't want you to do it alone.

When you have a bad day, do you call your personal trainer, celebrity pal, or private chef? Not if you live in the real world, Baby! You get on the horn to your best friend, favorite co-worker, or helpful neighbor. So, when you're ready to deal with the most personal journey that an overeater can take, why are you reading a book by someone who's slept at Buckingham Palace?

We are just like you. We've searched for happiness at the bottom of a bowl of Ben & Jerry's, we've lost weight all summer and gained it back all winter, we've eaten healthy foods all day and then binged all night.

This may not be the right book for you. Perhaps you enjoy the instability of the binge-purge cycle of the yo-yo dieter. Perhaps it's actually fun for you to wake up every Monday morning with a renewed commitment to weight loss and healthy living—only to find yourself inhaling an entire box of Oreos (in secret, of course) by the time Monday evening rolls around. Maybe it's better to bathe in the solace of the self-loathing that you know so well.

Or…maybe not. Maybe you're ready to take on a real partnership. Not the kind of joint venture that you've shared for so many years with Mr. Domino or Mrs. Fields, but an alliance where the partner gives back (something more than an extra roll of fat and one more notch on the bedpost of "best binges").

If you are ready to step into a world where healthy living feels more like a bonding experience than a torture chamber, then join us. The buddy system works. It's not a prescription with regulations and rules. It's just our story and we tell it with the hope that it will lend you and your friends ideas and concepts so that you can personalize your own program and begin a journey together to reach your own goals.

If not now, when?

In the following pages, we will provide you with the framework with which to build your own Healthy Lifestyle Program. Make use of our strategies, incorporate your own, learn from our personal triumphs and defeats as detailed in our later chapters. We share our stories (the spinning class successes and the sausage lasagna defeats) and thereby offer a guide to you on your own journey toward weight loss success. And by success, we mean not only pounds dropped, but vastly reconditioned eating habits and exercise routines, HIGHLY increased levels of self-esteem (I'm a princess! I'm a princess!) and a totally metamorphosed outlook on health, weight and the importance of powerful choices. Oh yes, and did we mention there were pounds lost? POUNDS! MANY, MANY POUNDS.

1 Weight Loss Plan, 2 Friends, 3 Weeks is a testament to the buddy system and how it can aid weight loss. Conventional wisdom tells us that it takes 21 days – 3 weeks – to form a habit. But this is not about science, nor is this a textbook. It's just our story and the strategies that we've learned along the way. We know this book can inspire and guide anyone who longs for a better body, a healthier life and a few laughs. Grab the hand of someone you love and start your journey together today!

Chapter 1

Finding a Buddy

Although we've only been writing this book for the last 12 months, we've been working on this healthier living/slimmer thighs project since the first day we met, over twenty years ago. Sometimes we were successful in our efforts, but our successes were always short lived.

Our plans were too complicated, our goals were unrealistic and our daily intake lacked moderation. Our plans were unbalanced; we neglected exercise or we congratulated ourselves for our brisk sprints around campus with jelly donuts.

We did discover that being accountable to someone was a big motivator, and so the plan we present in this book is based on that idea of teamwork and partnership.

We have found that using the buddy system fearlessly and ferociously is the key to living a healthier lifestyle. Choosing the right buddy is an important step in the direction of reaching your weight loss goals. In this chapter, we supply you and your Healthy Lifestyle Partner (HLP) with a list of

"Agreements" that detail what will be expected of each of you. Writing in your journal, staying in daily contact with your HLP, short and long term goal setting, and planning rewards for each other are all key factors in successful weight loss. We include a *1 Weight Loss Plan, 2 Friends, 3 Weeks* contract that you and your Healthy Lifestyle Partner can sign.

Are you up for this?

Before you make that vital commitment with a friend, it's important to ask your potential HLP some questions. It's no use working with someone who really doesn't have the time or motivation that you do.

Questions for potential Healthy Lifestyle Partner (and, yes, you have to answer them too):

- Are you up for this? No, really, are you really, really up for this?

- How much weight do you want to lose?

- What is a typical food day like for you?

- What exercise or movement do you do right now?

- Are you motivated by accountability?

- Will you still love me if I get irritable during this process?

- Will you remind me that this is a process and that negative thoughts should be shifted as soon as possible?

- Will you remind me to take this one day at a time and not self-sabotage by stressing about next week, next month, next year?

What are you willing to do?

Use your HLP for motivation. You are accountable to someone else now. Your success or failure is based on JOINT effort. So when you throw that alarm clock across the room and crawl back into your California King, you aren't just letting yourself down, you're letting your partner down as well. Check out these agreements and see if you can commit to a brighter lifestyle.

Agreements:

- We will contact each other by phone at least once a day.

- We will contact each other by email or text at least once a day.

- We will complete a list of goals and hold each other accountable for the actions that will help facilitate those goals.

- We will plan rewards for small victories and major wins.

- We will write in our journals every day.

- We will remember that we can't know how much weight we will lose, but we can be healthier and stronger every day.

- We will ALWAYS consult a doctor before starting any weight loss/diet/exercise/movement program.

- We will remember that we are each other's Healthy Lifestyle Partner and, whether you can hear a theme song or not, we are in this TOGETHER.

It may be very difficult to let go of your old bad habits as you begin this journey. It's hard to ignore your usual excuses for not making those healthy choices. So thinking of yourself as a TEAM, caring about the success of your friend, wanting her to reach her goal, even if you can't seem to see yours clearly in the moment, will help you put down the candy bar and head for the gym.

Healthy Lifestyle Partnership Agreement

_____ (hereinafter referred to as "me", "myself" or "I"), being of relatively sound mind and body, hereby agree and commit to the following Healthy Lifestyle Partnership Agreement (the "Agreement").

1.   I shall pursue a healthy lifestyle with the support of _____ (hereinafter referred to as my designated "Healthy Lifestyle Partner" or "HLP").

2.   Said pursuit shall be in reasonable compliance with the routine outlined in _1 Weight Loss Plan, 2 Friends, 3 Weeks, including but not limited to:_

- Daily morning check-in
- Daily accounting in my Healthy Lifestyle Journal
- Weekly weigh-in
- Trying something new each week

3.   I shall work towards the following long-term goals with the help of my HLP:

One month goal:
Six month goal:
One year goal:
Lifetime goals:

Healthy Lifestyle Partnership Agreement

4.   I shall hold my HLP and everyone else who may or may not provide me with input, support or annoyance during the performance of this Agreement harmless from all of my frustration, use of profanity and other means of letting off steam as I accomplish said goals.

_____
Signature

_____
Date

_____
Signature of Healthy Lifestyle Partner

_____
Date

Chapter 2

The Daily Plan

This plan will be a powerful inspiration to you as you begin this journey. By following a plan, you are focusing your brain on what it needs to do and not what it needs to eat.

Long-term goals (such as losing 20 pounds or feeling confident in a strapless dress) will motivate you. Short-term goals (such as eating more broccoli or attempting a boxing class) will be the core of your daily effort. It is important to create goals that are attainable and measurable. Chapter 2 will teach you how to set goals and create a tangible plan that will help you achieve them.

We're not going to tell you what to eat. You know what to eat. You say you don't know what to eat but you know that strawberries are a healthier snack than strawberry shortcake. Our plan involves getting you to do what you know you need to do: take action and be accountable.

Morning Check-In

Every morning, you will place a call to your HLP. *But I couldn't possibly talk to anyone before I've had 6 cups of coffee and a good loofah scrub!* Before you start in with excuses about why the morning is an inconvenient time to speak with your buddy, consider this: we have not just told you that every morning you have to do 3,000 sit-ups while chanting, "Thin is in! Thin is in!"

Calling your buddy in the a.m. will simply be one of many new habits you'll have to form. Like when you were three years old and you learned to brush your teeth every morning and not pick your nose in public.

This doesn't have to be a two-hour-what-did-we-just-talk-about-for-two-hours-conversation. This is your morning check in. The discussion need only include the following topics:

1) The Day's Eating Schedule
2) Strategies for The Day's Eating Schedule
3) Promise to your HLP

1) The Day's Eating Schedule
This is your chance to remind each other of what's happening in your eating world today. Are you heading to a breakfast meeting where donuts, Danish and muffins are plentiful? Have you packed a healthy salad and flat bread for lunch? Do you anticipate that this will be the evening when your other half decides

you should bond over a large pizza and bottle of red wine?

If you don't take the time to think ahead about how you'll incorporate healthy habits into your day, then you'll be an easy target for every Krispy Kreme advertisement and fast food drive-thru that happens to show up. At 3pm, it may seem like a good idea to purchase a Snickers Bar from the office vending machine; however, if you've already brought a protein bar for that crucial moment, you'll be sailing through those mid-day cravings.

2) Strategies for The Day's Eating Schedule

If you know that you'll be faced with a bakery bonanza at a breakfast meeting, you can lie down and accept defeat (getting up from the floor long enough to fill your purse with leftover bagels) or you and your HLP can strategize. This is your first food dilemma of the day, and surely won't be your last. Luckily, you're not alone. Your HLP won't endorse the idea that you are legally bound to ingest that coffee cake. Though you may try to rationalize the raspberry Danish as a serving of fruit, your HLP can stop you in your tracks with the suggestion to eat a healthy, filling breakfast before the meeting.

If you've already planned a healthy lunch, then your HLP can hold you accountable for eating that healthy lunch (rather than throwing the brown bag out the moment someone says "$4.99 All-You-Eat-Lunch-Buffet").

If your woman's intuition tells you that your significant other will want to confess his love for you over a carb-laden dinner, then your HLP can help you navigate that predicament as well.

3) Promise to your HLP

This is an important promise that ensures you start your day in a healthy living mindset. You agree to each other that you will stick to your plans and strategies for healthy living. You can use your own verbiage, or borrow from ours:

I promise to live healthfully today. If, for some reason, I feel that I want to use my body as a garbage can rather than a shrine to fabulous women everywhere, I will call you. I promise to do this for you, because if I'm going to be on track, then you sure as hell better be too.

Sometimes we add in extra promises that support the plan of the day. Whenever April goes out for Mexican food for a co-worker's birthday, she inserts, "I promise to enjoy the company of my friends, and NOT the entire basket of hot, greasy tortilla chips."

The Healthy Lifestyle Journal

It took us years, and lots of trial and error, but we've learned that keeping an account of what we eat, what chances we take and goals we set help us to always have clarity in our healthy living endeavor. And so, the major component of our program is…The Journal (or Diary, or Meditative Musing, or…)

With The Healthy Lifestyle Journal, you will write down your daily:

1) Food intake
2) Exercise
3) Daily Goal
4) Feelings/Stories/Victories/Moments of Hysteria/ Crises/Blunders

1) Food Intake

Perhaps you've tried writing down your daily food intake before. For the first three days, you scribbled down every meal with the commitment of a Jerry Springer guest trying to find out her Baby Daddy. If you ate a turkey sandwich, you even included the amount of mayonnaise and the number of sesame seeds on the bun. Over the next few days, you began to write less and less and suddenly, that extra cheese on your garden salad was conveniently unmentioned. By the end of the first week, you were tired of this little Home Economics lesson and decided that you would simply do a better job of remembering what you ate without actually getting your hands dirty with an ink pen. You likely stopped keeping a food journal because you weren't seeing the benefits of the process in a slimmer waist with every detailed diet confession.

Well, it's a beautiful new world out there and it's time to commit to writing everything down for this entire process! Don't do things the way you've done them before. You're better than that and your buddy needs you to stand up for her health as well as your own. So, if you eat it, write it.

2) Exercise

Is your partner working out three hours a day? Could that be excessive? Is she going for weeks without any physical activity? To lose weight, as we all know, we have to burn more calories than we consume. It's really that simple and we've known it for years. If you see that your partner is having difficulty fitting exercise into her busy schedule, help her to strategize. If she lacks motivation, be her cheerleader. If she's flying away from moderation and heading towards obsessive behavior, bring her back to earth. We're interested in changing our lifestyle in addition to our pant size, so we need to find calorie burning activities that we can realistically commit to in the long term.

What exercise are you going to schedule today?

3) Daily Goal

We all have long-term goals such as losing 30 pounds, or being able to walk a mile without feeling winded. You can include those goals where indicated on your Healthy Living Partnership Agreement. Long-term goals are excellent motivators - if you've ever taped a picture of a bikini-clad model to your refrigerator, you know what we mean. But that little bit of air brushed hope on paper never stopped us from grabbing a late night snack. Long term goals are too intangible. After all, summer is still four, five, six months away, right? There's always an excuse when you're thinking that far ahead, and it prevents us from focusing on the here and now. Daily goals are extremely important in that they require focus and dedication on a daily basis. Walk your talk – even if you're just taking baby steps. Daily goals can relate to exercise and food intake, such as promising to take a walk around the neighborhood no matter how draining your work day might be, or trying not to eat after 7:00 p.m. even though your favorite shows are on and sitting in front of the TV without a snack in hand feels akin to going to Disneyland and skipping the rides. A daily goal can be anything related to your quest for a healthier lifestyle, such as taking supplements or drinking the recommended amount of water. Whatever your daily goal, make sure it is attainable and measureable.

4) Feelings/Stories/Victories/Moments of Hysteria/Crises/Blunders

The food journal is an excellent way to help you start looking more like Wilma Flintstone and less like Barney Rubble; unfortunately, as with the Thigh Master you bought that hasn't felt the thrust of your thighs since you first opened the package, IT ONLY WORKS IF YOU USE IT. Keeping an account of food intake is a good start, but doesn't provide the satisfaction that The Healthy Lifestyle Journal can. We're going to ask you to put a little more of yourself into the daily record so that there's a little less of you at the end of each week. Not yet convinced? Try it for 3 days. Then stick at it for 3 weeks. You won't believe your mirror!

With our journal, you will see the benefits almost immediately if you set the journal up so that it suits your needs.

Option #1: Head to the nearest stationery boutique and buy yourself a beautiful journal for recording each day of this journey (no, a brown-colored spiral notebook made by Mead doesn't count). When you eat something, you can discreetly take out this gorgeous piece of literature and note what you've consumed.

Option #2: Document your day electronically. As you move through your day, you simply record the activities in a "draft" message that can be e-mailed later, or in a Microsoft Word document that can be printed out for your HLP. Quickly and efficiently, you'll make strides toward a better body through the use of 21st Century Technology.

Option #3: This last option is for the journal-phobic. Those people that just can't imagine taking pen to paper on a consistent basis. You can actually record your food intake in a small voice recorder/Dictaphone and replay the day's events as if you were Tom Cruise in Mission Impossible.

However you choose to record your day, the most important thing is that you do it honestly and consistently.

Journal Swap

Almost as fun as swapping stickers in the second grade and not as taboo as swapping husbands, you and your HLP will share your journals with each other every day. We have found that the best way to do this is by e-mail. Even if you are writing down every teaspoon of butter in your favorite Hello Kitty journal, it's easy enough to quickly type the info into an e-mail document and send it off to your HLP for review. If e-mail doesn't suit you, then you can always show each other your entries if you're lucky enough to see each other on a daily basis. It's also possible to call each other and give each other the good news (we hope!) that way.

Chapter 3

The Weekly Plan

<u>Weigh Yourself Once A Week.</u>

Before you begin this journey, you and your HLP should weigh yourselves and record your current weight on the first day of journaling. Does this suggestion cause you to foam at the mouth and howl achingly at the wind? Or are you the type that steps on the scale at every possible moment (even if it means digging Aunt Estelle's scale out of her bathroom cabinet and replacing it as neatly as possible before returning to the family's discussion of Wheel of Fortune contestants)? Could it be that you are actually the person who is standing on a scale right now—taking pleasure in the fact that this book weighs 2 pounds or maybe even 10?

We all seem to have a unique relationship with the scale. April loves the scale. She hangs out in the bathroom section of Bed, Bath, & Beyond and auditions every scale they sell. Don't be mistaken. She doesn't rejoice in what the scale often tells her. In fact, Stacey and any other amateur psychologist tell her that she uses her scale hopping as a means of punishing herself. Before April implemented the buddy system, she would allow the numbers on the scale to dictate whether or not she felt happy or slightly deranged. Did her obsession with the scale lead her to healthy living and that inner glow of (airbrushed, we remind you) magazine cover girls? Ha!

Stacey hates the scale. When she sees the numbers drop, she allows herself to loosen up on her healthy living lifestyle until a handful of chips becomes an entire bag. When she sees the numbers rise, she punishes herself in the same way. She has always preferred to let her clothes tell her when she's headed in the right direction. Loose pants mean pats on the back, tight skirts mean kick it up a notch. But you can ignore tight skirts for quite a while when you keep the top button undone. The numbers on the scale are far harder to ignore, and so, with support from April, Stacey has learned to brave the scale without falling apart.

Whether you weigh yourself yearly, daily, or hourly, we are pretty darn sure that you will have your own personal connection with that weighing tool that some believe was actually invented in the devil's workshop.

As much as we like the idea of you and your HLP weighing yourselves, hand-in-hand, as you sing a rousing course of "I Will Survive," it's best to weigh yourselves separately on the scales in your own homes. If you and your HLP plan to work out together in the mornings, then you can use the same scale. Although it's comforting to use the same scale, it's not sensible unless it is the scale on which you will always weigh yourself. Scales vary and we're less interested in the starting number than we are in seeing that number decrease over the coming weeks. If you start on your scale but then jump on hers at the end of the first week, we don't want to have to pick up the pieces when you discover that you haven't lost an ounce because her scale reads 2 pounds heavier than yours. (And the mystery of how you've weighed less than her all those years has been solved!)

There has been a lot written about the ineffectiveness of weighing yourself on a scale because of the information it cannot understand when you climb aboard. Does a scale realize that you are just days away from getting your period as it spits back a number you cannot bear? Can a scale take into account the fact that you haven't had a haircut in a long time and are therefore naturally lighter than it confirms? Will a scale ever be able to subtract the pounds that you carry when your heart feels heavy from a long day at the office? Not likely. But the scale can offer at least one measure of your efforts in the direction of weight loss. There are many other ways to measure your healthy lifestyle. Fewer inches, increased energy, and less food stains are all ways that you will be able to tell how well you're doing.

Every week, you and your HLP will record your weight in the Sunday journal. We chose Sunday because it motivates us to think twice before ignoring our long-term goal of healthy living and diving headfirst into a Saturday night pizza binge. Fun as that might have been in the past, we don't have to get our kicks from food in the same way anymore. We might even be able to recount some of the conversations we had that evening. If, as may happen with any of you over-achievers out there, you are dissatisfied with the number on the scale, you will be beginning a "No Excuses Monday" on the very next day. A "No Excuses Monday" mantra reaffirms our commitment to the plan whenever we feel we failed. No need for tears. Monday will sort you out.

Strategize for the Week Ahead.

Just as you strategize for the day, it is equally important to plan for the week ahead. Take a few minutes to discuss the coming week with your HLP. If you have a dentist appointment at the time when you and she normally walk together, you can find out if she is available for a morning stride. Perhaps she will tell you about an upcoming dinner date at an Italian restaurant where she would usually consume the entire bread basket before her fettuccine Alfredo arrived. As a team, you can plot a course for a triumphant week.

Try Something New Each Week.

Boredom can often lead to unhealthy choices. You know how it goes when you begin a diet. You're so convinced that you're the human version of Fat Albert that you're willing to ingest slimming chocolate shakes and low-fat crackers for the rest of your life if necessary. At first, the shakes and crackers almost taste good and you're sure that dieting has never been this easy or satisfying. But after a few days of the same foods, you begin to seethe at the thought of them. And so, not surprisingly, the very next time someone offers you Cool Ranch Doritos in lieu of those crackers, you eat so many that you can't even stand to be around your own chip breath.

It can be the same way with exercise. You find an aerobics class that you like and decide to make it your thrice-weekly cardio work out. That's great until, well, it's not great anymore. Maybe you'll eventually get bored doing the grapevine as you listen to the same Glee soundtrack over and over again. If you do the same exercises every time you work out, your muscles grow accustomed to the movements and you'll diminish the results that you deserve. This doesn't mean that every day has to look like boot camp. It's just important to think about the many ways that you can move to the groove of a healthy lifestyle, and we challenge you to raise the notch on your current level of activity.

The main thing to remember is that we want you to be successful. When you are choosing something to try this week, make it a winning choice. Although it's admirable to want to get past your childhood distaste for brussels sprouts, is it a good idea to eat them with every meal? Yeah, you're trying something new, but dare we say that you are committing healthy living suicide? Start slowly. When you read our journal entries in the following chapters, you'll see that there are many small ways to make a difference in your day. Maybe you'll like the idea of setting the alarm clock at the other end of the room and although you've considered doing this before, you'll commit to doing it this week. Perhaps you'll dive in and keep a bag of baby carrots at your desk like Stacey, or eat a turkey sandwich for lunch but leave off the mayo like April. We're not expecting you to finish first in a marathon by tomorrow, but we are expecting you to keep making the smaller adjustments that will keep you in the race.

Weekly Recap

- Weigh yourself once a week.
- Strategize for the week ahead.
- Try one new healthy living tip each week.

Chapter 4

Loving Your Body

Using a journal to communicate with your Healthy Lifestyle Partner will catapult you into living a healthy life. You will quickly see the benefit of keeping a record of your food intake, exercise and daily goals. Sharing your triumphs and failures with your HLP makes you accountable to each other. You will be able to better understand the other's specific weaknesses and struggles so that you can offer the best assistance and support. Chapters 4 through 11 detail some of our personal experiences as we used the Buddy System to change our lifestyles, lose weight and keep the pounds off for good!

Each of the following chapters deals with a specific topic (often common pitfalls for anyone trying to make healthier choices). After each example from our personal journals, you'll find tips that will help you to transfer the lessons we've learned to your own healthy lifestyle plan. These are detailed accounts based on shorter excerpts from our journals, so please don't think that the expectation is for you to write short stories to your HLP on a daily basis.

Sit back and enjoy a stroll through our own weight loss efforts...

Hi April,

I took a totally unnecessary stroll down view-my-own-ass lane today. As a negative body image experience, it rated somewhere between seeing a picture of myself squatting naked on the cover of a tabloid magazine, and getting on the scale after spending a week with my mother.

The setting: Major television celebrity's house. Or more specifically, major television celebrity's powder room, 1st floor.

My current job as an assistant event coordinator brought me to Mr. TV's beach side home. Excuse me, I mean "estate." I was planning his birthday party with his wife. As another negative experience, this rated somewhere between death (my own) and watching a litter of puppies drown.

The meeting went long. Very long. I had to pee when I arrived but the Mrs. wanted to get right to it, so it wasn't until three hours had passed that I finally excused myself to relieve the pressure.

I had seen the bathroom while we toured the house at a previous meeting. The mirrored walls made it look like the interior of a hotel lobby. This bathroom was larger than my bedroom, so vast in fact, that just glancing in from the hallway, I could not see beyond an enormous orange marble art piece displayed at the far end of the room. I was certain that if I walked past the sculpture I would see a line of 10 stalls.

As I excused myself, the Mrs. asked one of her house staff to assist me with the lights. (You know those wealthy folk can't just install a simple flip switch – much too common.) As her staff person turned on the lights and politely left me to myself, I began to make my way to the orange monstrosity in the corner. I had almost reached it when I realized that the bathroom didn't extend at all. It was the mirrors that had created the sense that the space just went on and on.

And that's when my foot hit the toilet. I walked right into it. It was chocolate brown to match the carpeting, of course. I reached out to steady myself and gasped. There was someone else in the bathroom with me. My heart raced as I recognized the hand I saw behind me as my own. The mirrors were everywhere and suddenly I had multiplied, my every movement mimicked by the hundreds of versions of myself that were reflected back. What was this? A bathroom or an immunity challenge on Survivor?

"Oh my God," I thought, "I'm going to get to watch myself pee." I mean, I could see myself from every single angle. Full frontal, full back, left side, right side, 3/4 left, 3/4 right and so on.

May I just say, I never knew my ass had such a personality. It was smiling, it was laughing, IT MOVED as I sat down (and every time I redistributed my weight once I was seated). I had no idea the jiggle capability of my behind. And seeing as how I'll never include it as part of the "special skills" section on my resume, I think I would rather have lived the remainder of my days without that knowledge and firsthand viewing experience.

I don't know how "close" you and your husband are in terms of sharing the bathroom, but my fiancé would pee in front of you and twelve of your best friends if he had to go and you were in his way. It's not my habit, but I have squatted in front of my man on a couple occasions out of sheer desperation. However, after today's adventure, I will invest in a box of Depends to keep on hand for future emergencies. Not only do I not want to expose anyone else to that vision of free-form flesh, but I hope that the trauma it has caused me does not resurface in dreams, waking me from my sleep, drenched in sweat, and begging, BEGGING for mercy!

Clearly, I did not enjoy being faced with how much weight I've gained in the last year. Clearly. But later this afternoon, driving home from the appointment, I thought about that image in the mirror and how womanly my shape has become - the curves and the dips and the softness. And I imagined myself, voluptuous and female, every bit a woman, surprising my husband-to-be with a very silly "come hither"

*dance in the neon light of our home office, with
nothing on my body but my engagement ring and a
flower tucked behind my ear. Not that I did that when
I got home, but I could imagine doing it, and how
thrilled my fiancé would be to see me celebrating
myself that way. I could live my life as that round,
curvy woman who loves food and cooking and eats
only things that taste "divine" and would never think
of touching a fat-free saltine because packaged food
lacks the "goddess quality." Wouldn't that be
something?*

Love,

Stacey

Tips for Loving Your Body:

1) Choose to love your body.
Instead of re-running her old fantasy about
how it would feel to be emaciated like a super
model, Stacey thought about inhabiting the
fleshy warmth of a pre-Raphaelite woman.
Since our brains can hold only one thought at
a time, why not make that thought something
positive? Stacey realized that she didn't
become totally satisfied with her body today,
but she opened a conversation with herself
about what's fine about her behind. This is a
much more fun topic of conversation than our
old standard, "Things That Suck About My
Body."

2) Take positive action.

Stacey can make a date to work on her rear-end at the gym tomorrow (a date that a Healthy Lifestyle Partner can make sure is kept). If you're dissatisfied with something, do something that will change how you feel about it. (And, no, unfortunately, consuming a large box of Junior Mints doesn't count.)

3) Get to know your ass.

It's also time to get to know your boobs. It's time to make friends with your flabby arms. And it's definitely time you asked your thighs to dinner.

Right now. This moment. You have a butt that's begging to come out and play. Check yourself out in a full-length mirror. Once you get past the negativity that will inevitably fill your mind, think about what you DO like about that rear-end. Does it smile like Stacey's or offer advice like April's? Does your butt like to take charge the way our friend Shari's ass does? Or is your derriere given to sexy pouts like our friend Olivia's? Find out.

4) Take it one day at a time.

Every day, you can challenge yourself to rediscover parts of your body. You can keep up this conversation with your bottom until you've made a truce with that giggling, jiggling flesh. Who knows? Your tush might end up being a good friend…the kind of friend who will definitely follow you on this journey to a healthier, happier you.

Chapter 5

Exercise

Taking those first steps toward exercise will be all-important in creating the healthy person that we know you can be. Even a little bit of movement is better than NO movement. Whether you choose to walk for 20 minutes with your Healthy Lifestyle Partner, try out a local aerobics class or jump rope in your apartment, you must celebrate every step you take!

While Stacey and April are good at flogging themselves for any and all dietary mishaps, they are equally adept at rejoicing in any and all actions toward healthier living.

Dear Stacey,

We are so good. We are so hot. I want to have sex with both of us! Look at what a fabulous day you had yesterday! Look at what a fabulous day I've had today!! I'm sure we must be the rock stars of healthy living.

My first day at the gym. My first day at a spinning class. Experiencing a range of emotions…

...total and utter love for you because our agreement with each other is the only reason that I got out of my warm bed this morning.

...total and utter disgust for you because our agreement with each other is the only reason that I got out of my warm bed this morning.

...joy at my ability to keep up with the rest of the class.

...anxiously competitive with everyone in the room--from my own husband (who cycles like a Tour de France competitor) to the gymnast on the bike in front of me (whose tush was smaller than the bike seat--oh, yeah, she needs the workout).

...running commentary inside my head about the instructor and how many thousands of ways she could be more motivating, better at explanations, kinder to new class members, and certainly keener about what kinds of songs would get my ass moving at 6:30am (Have you ever tried to sprint on a bike to the intro of "Lucy in the Sky with Diamonds"?).

As with all 45-minute periods of gym time, I felt the best when it was over. I was cocky, I have to admit, and I thought my husband, Nick, would be wildly impressed with his new wife's prowess in the spinning room. As we exited from my spinning class victory, what do you think Nick said to me?

"Have you seen your face? It looks like somebody spray-painted it red."

I mumbled something about how blood rushes to my face when I work out hard. I don't remember the rest of the conversation because I was immediately transported back to 4th grade P.E. when Dylan Dodson yelled across the gym, "Look at April-May-June! It looks like a cherry threw up on her face!"

No matter what demons may reappear from childhood, I am committed to this healthy lifestyle and I am committed to you.

Looking forward to hearing your report.

Lots of love,

April

Tips for Adding Exercise or More Exercise into Your Life:

1) **GO TO THE GYM!!!!!**
   April did. So can you. After all those mornings of hitting the snooze button, thinking she was doing herself a favor by allowing her body that extra hour of sleep, she did her body a REAL favor and got it moving.

2) **Try something new.**
Try a spinning class instead of sticking with your well-known treadmill routine. Venture outside your comfort zone to explore the vast world of cardio.

3) **Fuel yourself.**
No, it won't change the fact that you'll sweat like Uncle Arnie or turn bright red like April, but if you are going to exercise in the A.M., you need to make sure that you give your body the nutrients it needs. That doesn't mean bacon and a chocolate muffin—discuss with a nutritionist what foods will help your body stay satisfied.

4) **Tell the voice in your head to take a hike.**
Literally. If you're just starting out at the gym, you'll probably come up with several reasons why you should be doing anything other than aerobic activity. (Alphabetize the medicine cabinet, perhaps?) And it's okay to have these resistant feelings as long as you're having these feelings while simultaneously getting yourself moving at the gym or park or pool, etc.

5) **Use your Healthy Lifestyle Partner for motivation.**
Give your friend the best gift you can possibly give them: support for their good health. Even if you don't feel like dragging yourself out of bed, spring out of bed for the health of your

friend, your buddy – your partner in nice crime.

6) **Call your Buddy immediately for support when support is needed most.**
   If you notice the great should-I-or-shouldn't-I-workout-debate sounding off in your head, grab the nearest phone and call your HLP. Granted, you probably won't hear what you want to hear – "Yeah, you really should just take it easy in front of the television with an entire Entemann's Double Chocolate Cake". But then, you really don't want the weight loss results you've had in the past either, do you?

As always, please consult a doctor before starting any exercise routine or choosing how to fuel your body. Did we mention that we're NOT doctors?!! We're a lot of things, but we're not medically-trained.

Chapter 6

Self Image

Is anyone familiar with this dance craze? It's extremely popular and it's been around forever. I learned it from dear old mom. It's done without music or a partner and it's called "I'm-trying-to-find-something-to-wear-to-dinner-or-the-meeting-or-the-wedding-or-the-theater-and-not-one-single-item-of-clothing-fits-me." This dance is often performed in front of an open closet and ends with you and everything you own in a sweaty and scattered heap on the floor. Ah, so you've heard of it?

During this journey to a slimmer and healthier physique, it's important to adorn ourselves with clothing that makes us feel great. Beautiful. Special. Hiding in those oversized sweatshirts will not inspire and motivate. We cannot cocoon ourselves and play invisible as we wait for a transformation to occur. We need to love ourselves during this process by treating ourselves as if we are already slim. Eventually those pants from last year WILL fit again. In the meantime, it's important, though not always easy, to find something else that will...

Dear April,

There is nothing worse than walking into a department store in March, passing the newly set up bathing suit display and remembering how for the last 6 years you made a promise to yourself NOT to suffer through another fat summer and yet, here you are. No, there's nothing worse than that. Except of course, having to try on those bathing suits. But we won't get into that without several Xanax and a large bottle of Denial.

I was on a mission to buy. Sent by God, my fiancé and our satanic therapist, I was to update my wardrobe with size 12's and stop waiting until I dropped down to my natural weight of 102 pounds (always a dreamer) to replace the sweat pants (I love you sweat pants!) I'd been living in for the past several months. Golly, I don't know why anyone would see that as unhealthy!?

All day long I'd employed visualization techniques to garner strength for my expedition. I envisioned myself at the mall, trying on outfits designed specifically to enhance my larger bosoms and hide my wobbly thighs and flabby ass. I pictured suits for work, jeans, sweaters, boots and lingerie, skirts, dresses, scarves and hats. I looked fabulous.

At 5:30 p.m., exhausted by a long day at work, but determined to create a reality from the daydreams in my head, I decided to hit a designer discount department store/warehouse, overwhelming to most women, but a playground for this serious shopper!

Halfway to the store I began to perspire. I thought not of the fun to be had, but remembered instead the harsh light of the dressing room – one of those huge one-room dealies where all the women get naked together and try not to look up too often.

I suppose I should have paid attention to the droplets of sweat pouring down my forehead and onto the steering wheel. Perhaps I wasn't quite ready for such an adventure – especially after skipping the gym all week. But I ignored the signs. I heeded no warnings. I persevered.

I spent an hour and a half trying not to look at myself in the mirror as I tried on jeans, slacks, sweaters, skirts, blah de blah de blah. At one point, I had on a pair of tan work slacks. In the fluorescent light, I could see quite clearly the lumpy bumpy saddlebag cellulite. The woman trying on clothes next to me said, "Those look really good on you". She was in her mid-forties and sweet looking, with thighs that looked at mine as if to say, "Hey friend. I know you. What's shaking?"

I wondered what my face must have looked like that prompted her to encourage me with such a nice lie. It must have been a look of utter self-hatred. I was very upset. I left with three pairs of socks, and sandals that I won't be able to wear for another four months until the summer. I felt like a big fat failure and I ate dinner accordingly.

Some days, there is no past, there is no future. There is nothing except your butt-white bulbous thighs, and your saggy, flab-happy grandma arms.

The final lesson learned here, boys and girls? Communal dressing rooms suck and my therapist is the devil. (Yes, never look inward, as there is always somewhere else to place the blame!).

Hugs,

Stacey

Tips for Self Image:

1) **Shop for clothes in your current size.**
   Stacey's intentions were admirable. Even if prodded by her fiancé and therapist, shopping for some new things in TODAY'S size was obviously something that Stacey wanted for herself, as evidenced by her fantasies and the effort she put in at the department store. Life does not stop for those of us who want to drop 5, 10, 15 or 60 pounds. Activities and events continue to come up in our lives while we are still beginning our new journey--long before we hit the magic number on the scale or slide easily into those jeans from 2002.

2) Don't dress yourself in a cross between a Ninja warrior costume and a muumuu.
Dressing "FAT" (i.e. dark colors, oversized sweaters, sweatpants, etc.) doesn't hide anything--not from others, and more importantly, not from ourselves. When we look good, we feel good and when we feel good we look good. Get the idea?

3) Focus on the positive steps you take in a day.
There will always be nasty, horrible, downright sick things that happen, but why keep going over them in your fragile head? That's lunacy!

We all need to remember that once they add up, baby steps will one day equal a gigantic leap, and as long as we're moving in a positive direction, we need to give ourselves a pat on the back and a really BIG break!

4) Put some make-up on.
Dress yourself in cute shoes and a kitsch hair tie. There is no liposuction machine in your bathroom this morning but there is a basketful of different lipsticks and fun eye shadows that will make you feel...brighter.

5) Have a jewelry swap party.
Have you ever had one? They're so much fun and they net you some new stuff to make yourself feel different, new and covered in

bling. Each participant brings 2 or 3 or 10 pieces of jewelry that they like (none of the crap stuff) but that they don't wear anymore. Place all the jewelry out on a table like a fine department store. Choose numbers out of a hat to decide who gets to choose first. Let the swapping begin! Bracelets don't make us look fat. Widen your jewelry collection today.

6) **Say no to perfection.**
   It's much easier to live in a world that's either black or white; your choices are limited to two. This is good, this is bad, there is no in between. But those of us who've spent a lifetime in that colorless world know that it only invites disaster. We've got to be tough, determined, directed and driven. But to operate within such strict rules and regulations, whether self-invented or dictated by the most recent fad diet, is not the way to live healthy for the long term. As we first step into this New World full of endless possibilities, the ups and downs may be more frequent, but they'll be much less drastic. We have to allow ourselves the peaks and valleys. To deny that there will be meals of fat-laden, defibrillator-calling food, lazy days on the couch, and horrific shopping expeditions, is to assume that perfection is attainable. And people, that is just not the case.

Chapter 7

Mothers

Maybe your mom is skinny. Maybe your mom is plus-size. Maybe your mom thinks that you are skinny. Maybe she thinks that you are plus-size. Perhaps she told you that you shouldn't eat this or that you shouldn't eat that. Or maybe, she told you that you are perfect just the way you are.

This chapter can't begin to define the complexity of the mother-daughter bond. It's just helpful to notice the way that Momma has influenced the way you feel about cabbage or Marshmallow Peeps.

Remember! We're adults now, so whatever our moms have imparted to us about healthy living, it's up to us to take the helpful hints and throw out the impractical ones.

Stacey,

Ahhh...a visit to Mom's...the warm hugs...the unconditional love...the free chocolate. Am I alone in this mother-food connection or does being with your mom trigger the sudden and voracious need for large amounts of mac & cheese, rice pudding, and the scraps along the side of a bowl of cookie dough? Perhaps Dear Old Mom represents comfort and love (which, in adulthood, equals potatoes and pizza). Maybe Dear Old Mom rewarded me with one too many visits to Mickey D's during my formative years? Or possibly Dear Old Mom has a way of evoking numerous emotions with just one look?

Maybe I eat when I'm with my mom because of tradition or anxiety or happiness or boredom or inner-child longings or the fact that my family members cannot engage in any kind of meaningful interaction without the aide of large plates of fried food. Or maybe, just maybe, I eat a lot of food when I'm with my mom because, well, she's always offering me a lot of food.

But this time would be different. I live a healthy lifestyle now. I don't need the former trappings of the Jelly Belly filled candy dish. My cunning plan: Offer to make a healthy dinner for the folks. My mother was ecstatic about the idea (or so I thought). She said that she had no idea that I knew how to make vegetable risotto-what a clever daughter she raised! I was feeling good-approval from my mother while still sticking to my new lifestyle. This healthy living is a cinch.

As soon as my stepdad arrived home from work, my mother exclaimed, "I know! I know! Marcus, let's take April out to that new barbeque restaurant!"

April: I thought I was going to cook for you.

April's Mom: Oh, Darling, you don't want to do that! Wait until you taste the Buttermilk Biscuits at this place!!

April: (pause) (Thoughts of Buttermilk Biscuits.) (pause)

April's Mom: Unless of course YOU don't want to go out for barbeque! It's up to you of course, Darling! It's really delicious, though! Tell her, Marcus!! It's really delicious!!!

Marcus: It's really delicious.

And it was delicious. I was paralyzed by the menu though. How could I choose something healthy when my emotional torment levels were at an all-time high? Me, thinking that my mom doesn't trust me in the kitchen. Me, thinking that my thighs will be double-wide by the time I've sufficiently inhaled the Buttermilk Biscuits. Me, ovulating and therefore thinking that the "Biggie Brisket Basket" wouldn't be such an unwise choice. Me, thinking about the joys of family.

I did make it through though. Oh, yes, almost to my disappointment--I will admit to you. You know how it goes, you think, "well, if there's nothing to order but mashed potatoes and corn bread, I guess I'll have to be a good sport." But it was actually quite easy to make healthy choices because it was one of those buffet lines where I could see the food options (and imagine how they might look on my rear).

And, later, when my mom offered to make me a banana split with my favorite marshmallow sauce, I declined. I did however enjoy some frozen yogurt ("I don't know how long that's been in the freezer, April. Are you sure you won't let me make you a sundae or something?"). Again, I declined...happy to settle into a quiet, healthy evening with Dear Old Mom.

xoxo,

April

Tips for Handling Mothers with Care:

1) **Life is uncertain.**
   If the milk you had planned on having with your Special K is sour, should you opt instead for a half dozen doughnuts on your way to the office? I think not! Surprises are surprises. The unexpected will occur. We always have options within options. April realized that the way to handle her family time was completely up to her (and not her mom!).

2) **Though life may be uncertain, mothers are usually predictable.**
   If your mom is known for handing you piping hot homemade cookies the minute you walk in the door, be prepared. It sounds crazy, but

practice saying, "No, thank you." "None for me, thanks." "No!" And as much as you're able to talk about your weight issues with your mother, prep her in advance of a visit or dinner out. Let her in on your new plan – maybe she'll even offer to be your HLP! Maybe she won't understand or will disapprove. In that case, preparing yourself mentally and emotionally is just as important as keeping your hand out of her candy bowl. Create a powerful mantra and repeat it over and over on the drive to her house. Yes, it sounds ridiculous, but there are going to be times when your HLP won't be there to help you and forces are too great going against you to just "wing it".

3) **Laugh.**
   Love her. Forgive her her sins, for she knows not her effect on you, and likely your eating habits (good or bad) and your self-confidence, or lack thereof. You aren't fourteen anymore, she's not the enemy and you are your own person. Excuse her overbearingness or lack of interest or whatever it may be, and take control of who you are and what you want – in everything.

Chapter 8

Parties

While most people would be thrilled to receive a party invitation, you and your HLP may find that festive events challenge your Healthy Lifestyle efforts. Party fare doesn't often include soy milk and health bars. When Stacey headed out to a party with good intentions and lots of HL strategies, she found herself sideswiped by an overzealous hostess.

Dear April,

And the lesson learned today (one which I should already know by heart)....

So there I was, home from a loooonnngggg day of work, but gearing up for a going away party that I felt I just HAD to attend.

And so, I began the half-hour drive to Santa Monica. For the first three minutes, I drove in complete blackness with my headlights off. Yes, I was tired. So tired in fact, that the knowledge of my host's sick and twisted need to feed those who visit with a lust matched only by my always-working-overtime-

Jewish-mother, didn't scare me at all. Even though I had NOT been to the gym that day and even though I HAD indulged in leftover pizza for dinner. The Stacey of last year, or yesterday if you really want to get technical, would have used this social function as the perfect excuse to let this not-so-perfect day go to shit. But today's Stacey just wanted to laugh with some friends and then get to bed as soon as possible.

I was the first to arrive. Jenny greeted me warmly at the door and immediately ushered me into her dining room. It was the very scene I had imagined in my mind - a table laden with grapes and French bread, dipping oil, fresh cheeses and gourmet crackers. I was offered wine or beer, but with my eyes already closing, accepted a cold glass of water instead. We were having such a great time catching up with each other that I didn't even consider the food staring me in the face. Soon my buddy Dave popped in. We sat together and talked as Jenny continued her preparations in the kitchen. As Dave picked at the hors d'oeuvres, I began to pick as well. Was this habit? Did I just want to belong? Was Dave a dull conversationalist? I picked, but picked smartly - a few grapes, a couple of crackers - ABSOLUTELY NO cheese or oil.

Soon others arrived and the group was moved into the living room. I sat facing the coffee table, on which sat a bowl filled to the brim with nuts. I had to have a taste. "It's the good fat. It's the good fat." I kept telling myself. No guilt. Possibly a little piggish grabbing (I lost a few almonds down my blouse), but not out of control. And mainly, I was enjoying the company.

I was trying to figure out how to introduce the subject of my leaving. The party had really just begun, but it was starting to get late and I was focused on the 5:30 a.m. waking I had in store for myself the following morning. My very first session with the gym trainer! And then the words, well, word actually.....

"DINNER!"

I looked up and there it was. Where before there had been only grapes and bread, now sat a feast of sausage lasagna, homemade garlic bread and salad.

Shit.

I was still full from my dinner of leftover pizza. I had managed the party snacks without berating myself for having something other than fat-free cottage cheese and lettuce. I was at peace with my diet. I was still in control.

She came out with two plates piled high with food and tried to hand one to me.

"Oh, no, I can't ...I, no, really, I..." my voice trailed off as she interrupted LOUDLY with, "You're not having ANYTHING to eat??!?!?!?!?"

I was dumbstruck - a deer in headlights. I was Rainman, only I made even less sense, "I, uh, no, I uh, no, I um...I'll just grab a little something myself."

Jenny, again, so very like dear ol' mom, chose not to hear me and insisted on bringing me a "smaller" plate.

The second plate she brought me looked exactly the same as the first - well, no, there was only ONE enormous piece of garlic bread instead of two. How thoughtful of her.

So, here was the moment of truth. And how do you think I responded? Why yes, of course I inhaled the entire plate in five minutes flat, devoid of any enjoyment, waited an acceptable 15 minutes and politely excused myself from the evening.

And so, an apology to my mother. It's not you, it's me. I suppose my need to please exists beyond you, Mom. And I suppose, after spending the entire night half-sitting, half lying down and overwhelmed by nausea, I might be a step closer to learning how to survive this fatal flaw of mine.

Kisses - S

Tips for Partying:

1) **Eat before.**
   Eat a healthful, filling meal before you attend any event so hunger pangs don't make you inhale the buffet.

2) **Announce your intentions to the hostess at the beginning of the evening.**
   If you've already eaten, tell her as soon as you arrive. This will go down a little easier if you also make a remark such as, "Did I come to the right party? This looks like the work of Martha Stewart!"

3) **Strategize.**
   Strategize. Strategize. Make a plan with your Healthy Lifestyle Partner. Stick to it.

4) **Be accountable.**
   Set up a time to call your HLP and report on how you fared at the party. Just knowing that you have to recount your food and beverage intake will make you think twice about that handful of party nuts.

5) **Drink water.**
   Fills you up. Gives you something to hold. Makes you have to go to the bathroom (a quiet place where you can reflect on how well you are doing at the party).

6) **Focus on the other guests.**
I generally like to think that world revolves around chocolate and me; however, I know that this is not exactly true. Rather than day-dreaming about cubes of cheese, ask someone their opinion about world affairs. Engage in light banter. Lead a sing-along. The party will be a lot more fun if you enjoy the people around you.

7) **When you get home, write in your daily journal immediately.**
Do not stop. Do not pass go. Do not turn on a crime drama. Write down everything you ate. You're less likely to forget the globs of French Onion Dip that went with the celery sticks.

8) **Don't give up.**
There were many ways that Stacey's evening could have turned out differently, in both directions. She did a lot of things right. And she slipped up a little too. But, as long as she is willing to continue this wild ride called "Healthy Living - Even When You've Had a Childhood Like Mine", then she WILL succeed. The only way that she can fail is if she allows last night to mean DISASTER rather than EVENING-OUT-WITH-FRIENDS-WHERE-I-ATE-A-SECOND-MEAL-OF-LASAGNA-AND-THAT-WASN'T-PART-OF-MY-HEALTHY-LIVING-PLAN.

9) **Practice makes perfect.**

I know what you you're thinking. You think that if you were writing this book, you would tell Our Stacey to show more grit with hostesses and NEVER feel forced to eat. And advice such as that is legitimate. But does it really tell Stacey (or any of us) anything that we don't already know? We know we shouldn't take a second helping of Grandma's kugel just to make Grandma feel good, but we do. We know we shouldn't allow drinks out with friends to turn into buffalo wings and unpronounceable (but highly fatty) tapas consumption, but we do. And we certainly know that we shouldn't allow a hostess-on-a-mission to deter our own hard work and personal convictions, but we do. You, me, Stacey - we are all LEARNING. And we are all going to have to endure many, many evenings like the one Stacey endured last night, before coming to a place of peace with such an evening. We have to throw out the go-along-to-get-along mindset. And I hope you can understand that it is going to be with this practice, practice, practice that will allow all of us to get better at doing what's right for US and not the hostess, the grandma, the boss, the best friend, the cute guy, or the MOTHER!

Chapter 9

Saboteurs

Saboteurs may be those people with whom we share our lives, our hearts, and, on frequent occasions, our food. Parents, siblings, boyfriends, husbands, partners, friends and co-workers have a consistent impact on our daily routines; therefore, they are an integral part of our Healthy Lifestyle success. However, binge eaters are often embarrassed by the choices that they make or have made in the past. It is sometimes difficult to share our struggles even with those we hold so close.

Communication will be key in introducing these folks to your new Healthy Lifestyle. If you don't let them in on what you're trying to accomplish, they can't be blamed for suggesting Burger King or bringing home Cocoa Puffs in bulk. In addition, even when you do share what you need from your significant other or close friends, they may not be able to keep up with ALL of your idiosyncrasies. Be patient as you teach them how they can best support you, be brave as you share your struggles, and be strong as you take control of your weight, your health and your well being.

Yes, there are people we may come across, who, for whatever reason, make deliberate attempts to thwart our efforts. The ones that work at the mall offering samples as you walk by the food court are NOT out to get you. If you do encounter one of these, politely side-step them, but try not to do physical damage. Save your brute strength for slamming the door on the people you know personally, who get in the way of your making healthy choices.

Dear Stace,

Wanted to tell you about my snack today, as it was a bit unusual. It was not a protein bar or a nectarine or a bag of no-fat, low-calorie, vitamin-enriched chips of some kind. No, it was a brownie. A bar of rectangular chocolate that is as good for you as pouring an entire bottle of canola oil down your throat. So, you may be asking yourself, how did someone as healthy and health-conscious as April come to inhale a brownie? Well, settle in and I'll tell you a tale...

My birthday is tomorrow and I'm visiting my sister. A package from 1-800-Flowers arrived at my sister's house today. Elation flooded through me as I ripped open the box, imagining the long stem pink roses that might be inside. But instead of roses, I found a dozen gourmet brownies in every flavor imaginable—walnut, toffee, mint chip, white chocolate.

Unlike many people who would be thrilled by any gift, I was consumed by confusion and rage as I imagined beginning my 30th year with a dozen extra reasons as to why my thighs are so big.

Why is this happening to me?
What have I done to deserve this?
WHO would do this to me?

My skeletal sister, unaware of the total torment that I was now experiencing, asked me who I thought they were from.

I had no idea what monster had done this. It had to be from someone who likes me enough to want to pay the marked-up prices of 1-800-Flowers, but possibly someone who doesn't know me well enough to understand that giving brownies to an overeater is like handing out Piña Coladas at the Betty Ford Center.

I opened the card.

The brownies were from my own husband.

Why is this happening to me?
What have I done to deserve this?
Why would HE do this to me?

Just then, my brother-in-law walked in and asked where the brownies came from. My sister told him that they were from Nick. And the two of them had a 10-minute discussion about what a thoughtful man I married and how lucky I am that I have a guy who thinks ahead to shower me with gifts even before my birthday.

As much as I'd like to have a temper tantrum about the brownies, I know that they're right. I'm having an Oprah Light Bulb Moment and Oprah isn't even on for another 6 hours.

You see, Nick knows that I love brownies and I guess he thought I should have something that I enjoy as I celebrate the end of my twenties. And he's right. The brownies, my husband, my sister—are not responsible for my actions around chocolate. I am.

And let me tell you, the white chocolate brownie was scrumptious.

xoxo - April

Tips for Dealing with Saboteurs:

1) **Stay away from saboteurs.**
   As best you can. You may not be able to avoid them at the office but you don't have to invite them out for a mid-day coffee. Just to be nice. Being nice makes us great saboteur targets.

2) **Don't take it personally!**
   There will be times when people will make overtures that are not thoughtful at all, but it's unlikely in most cases that it's a calculated

and cruel plan to sabotage your efforts. They might be unaware of your struggle. They might be morons.

3) **Talk to them!**
   If the saboteur is your husband/mother/boyfriend/conjoined twin, talk to him or her. Really open up about what you're trying to do and what help you could use. People like to feel helpful. Can they stop by the organic fruit market on their way home? Can they help you cut up lots of vegetables and prepare healthy ingredients on Sunday afternoons to get you ready for the week? Are they willing to swap their love of food gifts for gifts of books they'd suggest? (Everyone likes to feel clever!)

4) **Be strong.**
   If someone offers you a box of illegal drugs, do you feel obliged to have just one hit to make the person happy? We hope not! Thank them graciously for their gift, dinner invitation or truck-load of baked goods and explain that you're feeling so good about being healthy that you won't have that/do that right now but appreciate their kindness.

5) **Don't make it about you!**
   So you've got a box of tempting chocolate from a not-so-thoughtful member of the public - deal with it. Eat it. Don't eat it. But don't make it about you. Just because your family

plans a party at a Mexican restaurant DOES NOT mean that you have to spend the evening with your hand permanently shifting between the chip bowl and the queso.

Chapter 10

Shopping

On this new journey to a healthier lifestyle we're not only overcoming poor eating and exercise habits, we're also updating and reinventing our sense of self. This includes throwing out the bulky sweaters (that do such a good job of slimming us down) and shopping for new clothes (that may not be the size that you will eventually be). Tough doesn't begin to describe the transition. Letting go of self-loathing and changing our attitudes about who we are, what we look like, and what we're capable of is painful. It takes courage, patience, and love. There are highs and lows as we shift our thinking and actions.

We encourage you to include shopping on your list of short-term goals. Perhaps you'll have an experience like Stacey describes below. Alternatively, perhaps you'll skip all that drama and still treat yourself to something nice.

Dear April,

There are bad people in this world. And these bad people, in addition to building nuclear warheads

*and destroying the rain forests, have created a
frightening world of push-up bras and g-strings. A
world of fishnet stockings and see-through teddies -*

VICTORIA'S SECRET

*My fiancé recently expressed disdain for the five-
year old sweatpants that I wear to bed nightly. And
so, as a promise to him, whom I love dearly, I went to
the mall in search of something sexy to wear. I was
determined to keep an open mind and was ready to
try on anything. Anything for $48.35, the amount of
store credit I had leftover from a Christmas gift gone
bad.*

*This particular shopping excursion to Victoria's
Secret was unlike any other, in that I had no choice
but to purchase something to slip over my dimpled
ass. After all, I do love James more than those sweat
pants. And so, due to the circumstances, a certain
amount of getting-naked-under-fluorescent-lighting-
stress was alleviated.*

*I took my time and browsed. I fingered fabric.
Dare I say it? I was ALMOST enjoying myself. I
gave an armful of options to the lovely 99-pound
employee, and stepped into a dressing room.*

*Oh the lights, bright and unbecoming, just as I'd
imagined them. But what was this? It seemed there
was a small space in the corner where if I faced the
Eastern wall and tilted 45 degrees forward, I could
completely avoid having to see my naked thighs in the*

three-way mirror. And as luck would have it, there also appeared to be an eight-inch space of darkness by the dressing room door where the dreaded lights didn't reach.

I quickly formed a plan. I would change with my eyes shut, jump into blackness and take a gander at myself through squinted lids. All this to avoid a panic attack surely brought on if I were faced with the reality of how much weight I had gained and how out of shape I'd become. Have you ever seen a grown woman stripped of her precious denial and left only with her lumpy white thigh flesh and extraterrestrial stomach pooch? It's not pretty.

Nothing seemed to fit. The tops were too loose or the bottoms too tight. I tried not be overly critical. I attempted to think of it from James's viewpoint, the viewpoint of someone who loves each and every curve of my naked body. So I didn't run screaming to the nearest Pizza Hut, but persevered. I went out to the floor for a second armful and returned to the fitting room with steeled determination.

It was getting late. The store was closing. It was do or die and I was not leaving the store without one of those idiotic pink and white striped bags.

In a moment of sheer panic, or brilliance, or both, I decided on a lacy black number with matching panties and took my place in line at the register. It was hot. I hadn't realized before how hot it was in the store. I mean, WOW. It was really sweltering. I lifted my hair off my neck and felt the sweat run down my back and soak the top of my pants. I tried to catch the eye of the girl waiting in line next to me.

"It's hot in here, isn't it?"

"No. I don't think so."

"Yeah, I swear they have the heat turned all the way up."

Perspiration dripped into my eyes as the impish salesgirl took my gift certificate. I thought I would pass out. I needed water. Water. Wow. You would think with the energy crisis, shops would be trying to conserve.

Or maybe it was just me.

xoxo,

Stacey

Tips for Shopping:

1) **Go shopping!**
   Yes, the first, mind-blowing tip for "Going Shopping" is to GO SHOPPING. Don't wait until you feel satisfied with your body. That's just an excuse to keep feeling miserable. If you curse yourself every time you put on jeans that are actually too tight, you can't possibly

start the day feeling good. How can you begin to reinvent yourself if you refuse to stop wearing clothes that make you feel like a beached whale?

2) **Take your HLP with you.**
   If she's not available (too busy whipping up a healthy barley stew), then take another good friend. You need someone there who will make sure that you don't spontaneously combust the moment that one of those chic sales ladies says, "Can I help you?"

3) **Promise yourself that you will try on no fewer than 4 garments.**
   If you're going to get undressed anyway, you might as well give yourself some choices.

4) **Call your HLP if you need help.**
   She'll stop you before you ditch the shopping idea and head to the nearest KFC so that you can purchase a sexy fried number instead.

5) **Put on some lip-gloss before you head into the store.**
   If lip-gloss is not your style, make sure you wash your hair. Don't enter into a clothing store at 2pm on a Sunday when you're hung over and sporting your Mickey Mouse t-shirt. If you don't feel good about how you look when you start the shopping expedition, the store's mirror will take on a satanic quality—

managing to make you grow a third eye and hairy breasts.

6) **Buy something!**
Don't wait for the moment when the perfect Donna Karan rip-off is hung under a sign that says, "Buy Me. You'll Look Great in This." Treat yourself to something today even if it's a size or so larger than you may need in a few months. You will move closer toward your goal if you treat your body with respect. Today.

Chapter 11

Families

Being with family members can often generate the need-to-feed. Why is this? Could it be because our families have the unique ability to transform our rational, adult-selves into quivering 6 year olds? Possibly. But even if you haven't taken your inner child to hours of intensive analysis, we're sure that you will see hints of yourselves in us. The names and places may be different, but the experience of family is often the same.

April recently spent a day with her family...the results were not disastrous, per se, just not advantageous for the healthy lifestyle that she's creating.

Stacey,

My mom and I are visiting my skinny sister in Georgia. Stephanie is the epitome of a hard act to follow—from the perfectly manicured nails to the size 2 (designer) skirts. I've spent the better part of my youth trying to (literally and figuratively) fit into her jeans.

Were I hanging out with either my sister or my mother individually, I would be singing praises of our tight bond and incredible ties. However, the combination of the two of them seems to ignite an insanity in me that can probably only be cured within a re-birthing therapy of some kind.

Being temperamental in the presence of my mother and older sister at the best of times, I found myself feeling like the third wheel in the happy reunion of first child (Stephanie) and first child's mom (Mom). We went to the mall as a threesome, but I was sure that the TWO of THEM were laughing at my panty-line every time I turned away.

We headed into Old Navy and my mother said, "April, you can leave Stephanie and me here if you want to look around at a different store." (Pause. Reminder to Self: Do not be overly sensitive.)

My Train of Thought: WHAT THE #@!*% DOES THAT MEAN, MOM? YOU DON'T THINK I DESERVE A $6.00 T-SHIRT BARGAIN? YOU THINK MY FAT ASS WOULD RIP A PAIR OF JEANS MADE IN THE SWEAT SHOPS OF CAMBODIA? WELL, THANKS, MOM, I GET THE SUBTLE HINT.

What I Actually Say: Okay. I think I'll go look for a Texas t-shirt for Nick (that wonderful man who loves me when no others do!).

Unfortunately, instead of finding my way to Tanya's T-Shirts, I ended up at Ye Olde Chocolate Chip Cookie Factory and before I knew it, I was buying a "Double Stuf" (cake icing stuffed between two large chocolate chip cookies which they spell incorrectly so you'll think about how cute it is rather than how fattening). Only problem was that I was standing in the middle of the mall with this Double Stuf! My mom and sister might turn the corner at any minute...finding me doubly stuffing my face!! Can you imagine what my sister would think?! Stephanie hasn't eaten a cookie since 2000! Naturally, I couldn't provide my mom and sis with more fuel for their family gaiety nor could I risk further humiliation by being caught with fattening food...so, what did I do?

Did I...Phone you for a reality check?

Did I...Remember to concentrate on positive images of my thin self walking confidently among a crowd?

Did I...Throw the Double Stuf in the nearest trashcan and march triumphantly back to Old Navy for grown-up conversation?

Ahhhh, shucks. Those are nice thoughts, but actually, it went more like this...I ate the Double Stuf in double time – barely allowing the cookie to touch the sides of my mouth before I washed it down with a Diet Coke (and a healthy dose of self-loathing).

When I went back to Old Navy, my sister threw her arms around me and said, "We missed you! Look at these bags Mom wants to buy us."

That was a temper tantrum that cost me 750 calories and 25 grams of fat.

Doesn't it feel good to get together with family?

Faithfully yours,

The Second Favorite

Tips for Dealing with Families:

1) Do a Reality Check

April wasn't thinking straight. She walked right into her familial situation with a lot of old junk taking up real estate in her head. Every look meant something negative and every spoken word was a direct comment on her weight. In reality, she should have been a little less narcissistic and a little more aware of what she was bringing to the table.

2) Talk about it!

If you can't get up the nerve to tell your mom that you want some attention too, then call your HLP and explain how you're feeling. Promise yourself that before you reach for a Double Stuf or a slice of Aunt Marlene's pecan pie, you'll get in touch with reality via your HLP. She'll be a much better listener than the voices in your head.

3) Strategize!
If you always end up foregoing exercise or eating too much around your family, make a plan for how you can react differently.

4) Take control!
If it feels like a punishment to listen to Uncle Dan's stories about how cute you USED to be, accept the family talk for what it is: diarrhea of the mouth. Don't punish yourself twice by using food as a quick hit of Valium. Now that really would be insane.

5) Self-acceptance and love is really the key to avoiding a Double Stuf every time you have to deal with family. When you really own those feelings, the "innocent" little comments thrown about so carelessly by Mom or Dad or Grandma will no longer send you running and screaming toward the nearest Dunkin Donuts. You'll just go running and screaming to no place in particular.

Chapter 12

Take the 3-Week Challenge

We are all on the same quest – to be our best selves. To let go of what was, even if "what was" was as recent as yesterday or even this morning. Live in the now. On this journey to healthier living, to a slimmer physique and increased self-love and respect, we must focus on the efforts we are making today, in this moment. To look too far ahead may be overwhelming and prevent us from taking control in the present.

<u>Tips for Gaining Perspective (so that you will embrace your best self!):</u>

1) **Volunteer.**
   Find a way to help someone else and you'll inevitably help your weight loss journey. How? Well, rather than thinking about what your next snack will be, you may start to focus on people who don't know how they're going to feed their children. Maybe, by volunteering in a place of need, you'll realize that some poor souls would love to have your problems. This isn't meant to be a lecture because we readily admit that we are vain, self-serving,

vacuous girls who would sell Grandma for a 28-inch waist but good things happen when we do good.

2) **Imagine your last days on earth.**
Imagine yourself on your death bed. Do you really wish you'd tried one more diet or will you be happiest at the thought of the wonderful people in your life? Do you want the happy memories of a lifetime of dieting – or the happy memories of a lifetime well shared with amazing people?

3) **Remember April's Mom.**
April's Mom had cancer for many years but her death came rapidly at the end. April rushed to the hospital to see her and blurted out, "You look great! So thin!" because April's diet-obsessed mind was actually pleased to see that her mother had finally shifted those last 15 pounds. What April didn't realize is that the weight had been lost within three days and was the sign that her mom was soon going to die. This is quite a downer of a story but it brings into focus how ridiculous our weight obsession is. After April complimented her mother on her thin physique, her mom smiled and said, "It wasn't worth it." April's mom died two days later.

4) Know the difference between perspective and excuses.

If you've seen the light and you realize that your ample hips are not actually at the top of most people's list of world problems, don't use that as an excuse to break out the chips. Use your new perspective to broaden yourself not your thighs.

So, take our 3-Week Challenge!

It only took us 3 weeks to know we were on to something good. Now, it's your turn.

1) Commit to 3 weeks.
2) Find an awesome friend to join you.
3) Follow the daily plan and watch the buddy system work its magic.

If all else fails, remember this:

Stacey & April's "Ate" Weighs To Eat Healthfully

OKAY, FRIENDS ... THESE ARE THE TOP THINGS WE KEEP IN MIND AND HOPE YOU WILL TOO...

1) **Put your fork down between bites.**
   Sounds easy enough, doesn't it? Well, do you actually do it? Of course not, because at first putting your fork down between bites is as easy as translating a medical textbook into Pig Latin. At first, we had a very hard time with actually putting our fork down between bites. It felt as if the moment we put our fork down, there was a small animal screaming out in pain inside of us until we could quiet it down by lifting up the fork again.

2) **Count your blessings not your French Fries.**

If we can take the time to think about all of the wonderful reasons that we want to live healthfully, we may be able to stop obsessing about food and start living the healthy lifestyle that will lead us to the richest life available. A life where we're focused less on when we'll be able to eat again and more on the incredible people and joy that surrounds each and every one of us. Take a moment to examine all of the reasons that you want to stay on track. Do you want to have more energy so that you can play with your children or dance with your friends? Do you have a responsibility to your boyfriend/husband/family/children to stay healthy and alive (leaving your poor habits and the risk of diabetes and other weight-related diseases behind)? Is it possible that you've been so busy thinking about what you're eating at parties that you haven't been able to enjoy the people there with you? Counting your blessings before/during/after eating is one easy, no-cost way to give thanks. One more slice of cake may seem harmless enough, but is it going to lead you to the kind of life that you've always wanted?

3) **Stop eating when you're full.**

While this is not a revolutionary concept, it is often the most underused and easiest weight loss tool available. Before you close this book and look for the magic pill, hear us out! This could mean as much to you as Stacey, who used to polish off a family-size bag of Lay's Potato Chips in one sitting. April used to order an entire pizza and eat every bite herself. Were we eating past the point of being full? Most definitely. Had we been eating to satiate our hunger, then we could have stopped with one serving (rather than 12). But, Ladies, as any overeater will tell you, we rarely eat a second piece of mom's pie because we're famished. Emotionally, we need more. Instead of lighting up a cigarette or snorting a line of cocaine, we're chomping on Famous Amos' finest because that's how we cope best.

Just as a non-smoker has a hard time understanding how people can continue with the filthy habit of puffing away on "cancer sticks," someone who doesn't habitually overeat will have a hard time of understanding why you can't just enjoy a little taste of birthday cake. The truth is that YOU CAN teach yourself to do just that. But you'll need the support of your buddy in order to train yourself to savor every morsel that your body wishes to consume.

4) **Don't let yourself go hungry.**
This doesn't mean that you should eat non-stop all day long. We simply believe that if you feel hungry, you should eat. Your stomach is growling for a reason. This is the

flip side to stopping when you're full because we've discovered that starving leads to misery and a large shopping spree at Dunkin Donuts. If you allow your stomach to get completely empty, you'll be more likely to binge out of frustration and temporary insanity induced by a dip in blood sugar. Keep a healthy snack on-hand for emergency munching.

5) **Practice moderation.**
Oooh! This one hurts, we know. The thought of not being able to stuff endless cookies and candies into your body (a "temple", right?) makes you feel more deprived than anything. Imagine how deprived you'll feel when you can't wear the dress that you love because it's too tight.

6) **If you think you're going to overeat, call your HLP.**

7) **Focus on the positive.**
We don't have to stand around holding hands, singing Kumbaya but we do have to stop pretending that a happy mindset is for hippies. It's always easy to get down on ourselves but focus on your tremendous effort! The worst part is (and ALWAYS is) that in our effort to treat ourselves well with healthy living, we feel we have to be perfect. If you punish yourself for falling off the wagon with more food, then you're an egg salad short of a picnic. No unhealthy dinner is nearly as bad

for our bodies as it is for our confidence and drive.

8) **Ditch your perfectionism.**
Not easy to do but totally necessary if you are the type of person that allows ONE donut to crush your dreams of healthy living. Don't be perfect. It's exhausting and it makes you less fun.

It's difficult to enjoy food when you're using it to either flog yourself for all your perceived flaws, or treating it as evil – every morsel equal to another mass of thigh cellulite. You will never reach your goal while treating food as Good or Evil. Exercise, eat your vegetables, avoid fried foods...but if hard and fast rules are made, then they can be broken. So allow yourself the treats. Enjoy eating again. Let go of the monotony of categorizing foods as "good" or "bad". Eat wisely, but eat what tastes good. Be satisfied. Be delighted. Food is not the enemy. You are your own enemy. Kill the negativity and the self-hatred and the nasty voice in your head that points out every imperfection, and you will succeed.

Engaging a Healthy Lifestyle Partner makes you accountable to someone else to be the best version of yourself. By using the buddy system, you each take the focus off yourselves and your wobbly tummies-- and start making changes that support one another. We've tried all of these techniques and they worked for us. We're not toting anything revolutionary here, just common sense. But sometimes, when we're really lost and things seem darkest, it's the basics we need to be reminded of in order to pull ourselves up and start fresh.

We have used all of the strategies in *1 Weight Loss Plan, 2 Friends, 3 Weeks* and they worked. We know they can work for you too!

Resources

http://www.choosemyplate.gov/
Check out healthy eating from the US government. In response to criticisms about the notorious food pyramid, MyPlate includes four food sections with a fifth section off to the top-right side. The MyPlate website also includes tips for staying healthy and how to incorporate these food items into your everyday meals. The addition of daily exercise is also a large part of the MyPlate program. Although we are not going to tell you what to eat, we think this is a good starting point as it's run through the USDA.

https://www.nationaleatingdisorders.org/
The National Eating Disorders Association (NEDA) is the leading non-profit organization in the United States advocating on behalf of and supporting individuals and families affected by eating disorders. Even if you don't have an eating disorder, this website is a helpful resource of information about living a healthy life.

http://www.bedaonline.com/
Binge Eating Disorder Association (BEDA) provides individuals who suffer from binge eating disorder with the recognition and resources they deserve to begin a safe journey toward a healthy recovery.

Things To Do With Your Hands
While Watching TV
(instead of sticking them in the cookie jar)

Doodle
Google
Clean out a junk drawer
Knit/Crochet/Macramé
Fold laundry
Make shadow puppets
Pen a love letter
Tweeze stray hairs
Give yourself a manicure
Give yourself a tattoo
Alphabetize books
Practice jazz hands
Rearrange the furniture
Solve complex equations
Pop bubble wrap
Polish the silver
Polish your shoes
Build a LEGO village
Lift hand weights
Levitate the cat
Deliver a baby

Scratch an itch
Pet a dog
Scrapbook
Knead dough
Organize files
Hammer a nail
Dribble a ball
Learn origami
Floss
Dissect a frog
Iron
Pay bills
Spin a dreidel
Finger paint
Dust
Chop vegetables
Play Jacks
Braid your hair
Cut your hair
Clip Coupons
Journal it out

Acknowledgements

Thank you to our amazing editors, Matt[2], for their suggestions, corrections and unwavering support. Without them, this book wood bee won phat mes.

Thanks to our Ithaca friends and professors for igniting our creativity.

Another thank you is due to all of our post-grad friends and mentors who have continued to inspire us.

Finally, thank you to our families, our parents in particular, for providing us the neurosis necessary to embark on this endeavor.

About the Authors

When April and Stacey met at Ithaca College, they fed each other's love of theatre, music and high fat foods. Their friendship reached dizzying heights when they discovered that, not only could you get pizza delivered to your dorm room, but also warm chocolate chip cookies with a side of milk.

April is a writer and teacher with a deep love of Van Gogh and a great fear of eye boogers. After a decade in England, she now resides in Texas with her husband and two children.

Stacey is a writer and artist with an appreciation for dark humor, which she explores in her developing cartoon series, Gynecopia. She lives in California with her husband and three children.

Both women married men named Matt.

www.ingramcontent.com/pod-product-compliance
Lightning Source LLC
Chambersburg PA
CBHW032029290526
45786CB00011B/1239